ONE TOUCH
NURSING
CALCULATIONS

Nursing Calculations Made Easy

SAM DJANIE

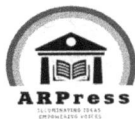

ARPress
ILLUMINATING IDEAS
EMPOWERING VOICES

ARPress
45 Dan Road Suite 5
Canton MA 02021
Hotline: 1(888) 821-0229
Fax: 1(508) 545-7580

Ordering Information:
Quantity sales. Special discounts are available on quantity purchases by corporations, associations, and others. For details, contact the publisher at the address above.

Printed in the United States of America.

ISBN-13:   Softcover   979-8-89389-548-3
             eBook   979-8-89389-550-6
             Hardback   979-8-89389-549-0

Library of Congress Control Number: 2021917150

CONTENTS

INTRODUCTION

This method is called the "Unit Cancellation Method" (UCM) It does not require us to know the many formulae of medication calculations which we oftentimes forget; at clinical settings and in exams. It is natural to forget formulae because we don't use them everyday and things we don't use everyday, we tend to forget. This process uses the numbers right in front of us to complete the calculation in no time; this is fun!

CONCEPT

LETS START FROM THE BASICS:

EXAMPLE 1: HOW MANY CENTS ARE IN 2 DOLLARS?

The first point to realize here is that, our final answer will be in cents, so we must arrange our problem in such a way that our cents will be up in the numerator.

ANSWER:

To be Given : 2 dollars

Relationships from Tables: 100 cents = 1 dollar

SET UP

TO BE GIVEN X RELATIONSHIP FROM TABLES

TECHNIC:

1) Pay particular attention here. In order to place cents in the numerator, because that's what we want, we can manipulate the relationship from tables, anyway we want.

2) THE GIVEN UNIT WANTED must be in the numerator. With these points in mind, we can tackle our problem now.

1

SOLUTION

$$\frac{(100\ Cents)(2\ dollars)}{(1\ dollar)}$$

(100 x2) cents = 200 cents

Example 2: How many cc(ml) are in 2L

ANALYSIS:

To be Given: 2 L

Our answer should be in cc so we put cc in the numerator.

TABLES:

We know that 1,000 cc(ml) = 1 L

WATCH CAREFULLY HERE

We will arrange the table relationship so that the liters will cancel and our final answer will be in cc(ml).

$$\frac{(1,000\ cc)(2L)}{1L} = (1,000 \times 2)\ cc$$

ANSWER = 2,000 cc

This simple principle runs through all medication problems.

ADMINISTRATION OF TABLETS

TWO STEPS PROBLEMS

Q1) The doctor's order says: Give 250 mg. The label says 0.5 Gm per tablet. You will give-tablets to the patient.

ANSWER:

Most questions in Nursing need 2 steps, so watch very carefully here, but we can represent every problem on one line. The first thing to note here is that, the amount of medication including its units to be given must be in the numerator. Another important thing to note is that tablet must be in the numerator since that's what we are looking for in our final answer.

STEP ONE:

The question says 0.5 Gm per tablet. This means 0.5 Gm = 1 tablet. This can be represented as 0.5 Gm/1 tablet

Or 1 tablet/0.5 Gm

The choice of which relationship we decide to use depends on what type of cancellation we want to do. No matter what we do, we will arrange this relationship so that the tablet will be in the numerator.

ANALYSIS

To be Given: 250 mg.

FROM TABLES: 1,000 mg = 1Gm

ANOTHER RELATIONSHIP ON THE LABEL: 1 tablet = 0.5Gm

Or 1 tablet/0.5Gm

So, our step one to this problem will look like this

$$\frac{(250 \text{ mg})(1 \text{ tablet})}{(0.5 \text{ } Gm)}$$

STEP TWO:

Our second and final step (or conversion) will make use of tables.

From tables, we know that, **1 Gm = 1,000 mg**

Which we can represent as 1 Gm/1,000mg or 1,000mg/1 Gm. Our choice will depend on what type of cancellation we want to do. We will arrange this relationship in such a way that we can do all necessary cancellations of units, so that we have tablet as our final answer.

STATEMENT 2:

$$\frac{(250 \text{ mg}) (1 \text{ tablet}) (I \text{ Gm})}{(0.5 \text{ Gm})(1,000 \text{ mg})}$$

$$\frac{(250 \text{ tablet})}{(0.5)(1,000)} = \frac{250 \ 1 \text{ tablet}}{500 \ 2}$$

1/2 tablet

Or

$$\left(\frac{1}{2}\right) \left(\frac{5}{5}\right) tab = \left(\frac{5}{10}\right) tab = 0.5 \text{ } tablet$$

How to Change Fractions to Decimals

QUESTION 2

The doctor orders Tylenol for Mrs. Brown's headache. The doctor's order says: Tylenol 650 mg PO Q4h PRN for pain. The label on the Tylenol bottle reads: 325 mg/tablet. How many tablets will the Nurse give to Mrs. Brown when she complained of headache.

STEP ONE

ANALYSIS

To be Given=Doctor's order=650 mg

Relationship: 325 mg/tablet

STEP TWO

$$\frac{\overset{2}{\cancel{(650 \text{ mg})}}(1 \text{ tablet})}{\cancel{(325 \text{ mg})}}$$

$$= 2 \text{ tablets}$$

So the Nurse will give 2 tablets to Mrs. Brown.

QUESTION 3

Mr Jones is hypokalemic and the doctor orders potassium tablets for Mr Jones. The doctor's order reads: Give 40 milliequivalent (meq) of potassium Stat. The label on the bottle reads: 20 meq/tablet. How many tablets will the nurse administer to Mr Jones?

STEP ONE

ANALYSIS

TO BE GIVEN:

DOCTOR'S ORDER: 40 meq

Relationship: 20 meq/tablet

STEP TWO

$$\dfrac{\overset{2}{\cancel{(40\ meq)}}\ (1 tablet)}{\cancel{(20\ meq)}}$$

2 tablets

QUESTION 4

The Doctor's order reads: Give lasix (furosemide) 40 mg PO Stat. The label on the medication tag reads 20 mg per tablet. How many tablets will the nurse give to the patient?

STEP ONE

ANALYSIS

TO BE GIVEN:

40 mg

Relationship: 20 mg per tablet

STEP TWO

$$\frac{\overset{2}{(\cancel{40 \text{ mg}})} (1 \text{ tablet})}{(\cancel{20 \text{ mg}})}$$

2 tablets

QUESTION 5

Mr Stephens has a history of hypothyroidism. The doctor orders Synthroid for Mr Stephens. The order reads: Give Synthroid 0.025 mg. The label on reads; .050 mg/tablet. How many tablets will the nurse give to Mr Stephens?

STEP ONE

ANALYSIS

TO BE GIVEN: Doctor orders, 0.025 mg

Label reads: 0.050mg/tablet

STEP TWO

$$\frac{\frac{(0.025 \text{ mg}) (1\text{tablet})}{(0.050 \text{ mg})}}{2}$$

$= ½$ tablet

MEDICATION ADMINISTRATION TERMINOLOGIES AND STANDARD TABLES

Abbreviations	Latin	Word Meaning
Ac ante	cibum	before meals
Ad lib	ad libitum	freely
am ante	meridian	morning
bid	bis in die	twice a day
c	cum	with
cc, cm	cubic centimeter	cubic centimeter(ml)
D/C, or DC	Discontinue	terminate
Elix	Elixir	elixir
Gtt	Gutta	drop
H, hr	hora	hour
Hs	Hora somni	at bedtime
IM	Intramuscular	into a muscle
L	Left	left
L	Liter	liter
Min or m	Minim	minim(1/15 or 1/16 ml)
O	no or none	no or none
OD	oculus dexter	right eye
OS	oculus sinister	left eye
Os	os	mouth
OTC	over-the-counter	nonprescription drug
OU	oculus uterque	each eye
Pc	Post cibum	after meals

PM	post meridiem	afternoon
PO	per os	by mouth, orally
Prn	pro re nata	as needed
Pr	Patient	patient
Q	quaque	every
Qd	quaque die	every day
Qh	quaque hora	every hour
Q4h, q4	every 4 hours	every 4 hours
Qid	quarter in die	4 times a day

QUESTIONS ON TABLET ADMINISTRATION

(ANSWERS WILL BE FOUND AT THE BACK OF THE PAGE)

1) Cecil had surgery yesterday and the doctor orders morphine sulfate for Cecil. The Doctor's order reads: Give morphine sulfate 20 mg PO Q4H PRN for severe pain. The label on the medication bottle reads: 10 mg/tablet. How many tablets will the Nurse give Cecil when she is in severe pain?

   A. 1 tablet
   B. 2 tablets
   C. 3 tablets
   D. 4 tablets

2) Mr Gerry is very anxious. The psychiatrist ordered Librium for Mr Gerry. Give Librium 30 mg PO BID for anxiety. Librium tablets are supplied as 15mg/tablet. How many tablets will the Nurse give to Mr Gerry at a time.

   A. 1 tablet
   B. 2 tablets
   C. 3 tablets
   D. 4 tablets

3) Mr. Jones is diabetic and the doctor orders Glucophage for Mr Jones. The doctor's order reads: Give Glucophage 1,000 mg PO OD. The Glucophage bottle reads: 500mg/tablet

    A. 1 tablet
    B. 2 tablets
    C. 3 tablets
    D. 4 tablets

4) The doctor orders klonopin for Mr. Stevens because Mr. Stevens is very anxious. The doctor's order says, give klonopin 2 mg PO bid PRN. Klonopin comes from the manufacturer as follows: 1 mg per tablet. How many tablets will the nurse give to Mr. Stevens at the time he is experiencing anxiety?

    A. 1 tablet
    B. 2 tablets
    C. 3 tablets
    D. 4 tablets

5) The doctor's order says, give colace 200 mg PO HS. Colace is labeled as 100 mg/tablet. How many tablets will the nurse give to the patient?

    A. 1 tablet
    B. 2 tablets
    C. 3 tablets
    D. 4 tablets

6) The doctor orders dalmane 20 mg for a patient to be taken during bedtime. Dalmane tablets come from the manufacturer as 10 mg per tablet. How many tablets will the nurse give the patient?

    A. 1 tablet
    B. 2 tablets
    C. 3 tablets
    D. 4 tablets

7) The doctor orders xanax 0.25 mg PO TID. Xanax comes labeled 0.25 mg/tablet. How many tablets will the nurse give to the patient?

    A. 1 tablet
    B. 2 tablets
    C. 3 tablets
    D. 4 tablets

8) The doctor's order says, valium, 10 mg PO BID. Valium is labeled 10 mg per tablet. How many tablets will the nurse give the patient?

    A. 1 tablet
    B. 2 tablets
    C. 3 tablets
    D. 4 tablets

9) The patient is experiencing some parkinsonian effects and the doctor ordered cogentin for the patient. The doctor's order says, Cogentin 1 mg PO Daily. Cogentin is labeled as 0.5 mg per tablet. How manty tablets will you give to the patient?

    A. 1 tablet
    B. 2 tablets
    C. 3 tablets
    D. 4 tablets

10) The doctor orders Robaxin for a patient as a skeletal muscle relaxant. Give Robaxin 2 Gm PO QID. Robaxin comes as 1 Gm per tablet. How many tablets will you give?

    A. 1 tablet
    B. 2 tablets
    C. 3 tablets
    D. 4 tablets

ANSWERS TO TABLET QUESTIONS

1) B

Doctor's order 20 mg of morphine sulfate.

On label 10 mg per tablet or 10 mg/l tablet or 1 tablet/10 mg Set up: (To be Given doctor's order)(Right Relationship)

$$\frac{\overset{2}{\cancel{(20mg)}}(1tablet)}{\cancel{10mg}}$$

$$(2)(1 tablet)=2 tablets$$

So, the nurse will give 2 tablets of morphine sulfate to the patient

2) B

Doctor's order: 30 mg of Librium

Supply Label: 15 mg/1 tablet or 1 tablet/15mg

Set up: (To be Given) (Right Relationship)

$$\frac{\overset{2}{\cancel{(30\ mg)}}(1\ tablet)}{\cancel{(15mg)}}$$

$$= (2)\ (1\ tablet)$$

$$= 2\ tablets$$

So the nurse will give 2 tablets of Librium to the patient.

3)   B

Doctor's order: 1,000 mg of Glucophage

Label inscription: 500mg/1 tablet or 1tablet/500 m;

Set up: (To be Given Doctor's order) (Right Relationship)

$$\frac{(\overset{2}{\cancel{1,000}}\ mg)(1\ tablet)}{(\cancel{500}\ \cancel{mg})}$$

2 tablets

So the nurse will give 2 tablets of Glucophage to the diabetic patient.

4)   B

Doctor's order: 2 mg of klonopin.

Label Relationship: 1 mg per tablet or 1 mg/1 tablet or 1 tablet/1 mg

Set up: (To be Given Doctor's order) (Right Relationship)

$$\frac{(2\ \cancel{mg})\ (1\ tablet)}{(1\ \cancel{mg})}$$

(2)(1 tablet)

2 tablets

So, the nurse will give 2 tablets of klonopin to the patient.

5) B

Doctor's Order: 200 mg of colace.

Label Relationship: 100 mg. /1 tablet or 100 mg/1 tablet or 1 tablet/100mg

Set Up: (To be Given Doctor's order) (Right Relationship)

$$\frac{(\cancel{200 \text{ mg}})^{2} (1 \text{ tablet})}{(\cancel{100 \text{ mg}})}$$

(2)(1 tablet)

=2 tablets

So, nurse will give 2 tablets of colace to the patient.

6) B

Doctor's Order: 20 mg of Dalmane

Label Relationship: 10 mg per tablet or 10 mg/1tablet or 1tablet/10 mg

Set Up: (To be Given Doctor's Order) (Right Relationship)

$$\frac{(\cancel{20 \text{ mg}})^{2} (1 \text{ tablet})}{(\cancel{10 \text{ mg}})}$$

(2) (1 tablet)

2 tablets

So, the nurse will give 2 tablets of dalmane to the patient

7)   A

Doctor's order: 0.25 mg of Xanax

Label Relationship: 0.25 mg per 1 tablet or .25mg/tablet or 1tablet/.25mg

Set Up: (To be Given Doctor's Order) (Right Relationship)

$$\frac{1}{\frac{(0.25 \text{ mg}) (1 \text{ tablet})}{(0.25 \text{ mg})}}$$

1

1tablet

So, the nurse will give 1 tablet of Xanax to the patient

8)   A

Doctor's Order: 10 mg of valium

Label Relationship: 10 mg per tablet or 10 mg/1 tablet or 1tablet/10 mg

Set Up: (To be Given doctor's order) (Right Relationship)

$$\frac{1}{\frac{(10 \text{ mg}) (1 \text{ tablet})}{(10 \text{ mg}) \, 1}}$$

1tablet

So, the nurse will give 1 tablet of valium to the patient.

9) B

Doctor's Order: 1 mg of Cogentin.

Label Relationship: 0.5 mg per tablet or .5mg/1 tablet or 1 tablet/.5mg

Set Up: (To be Given doctor's Order) (Right Relationship)

$$\frac{\overset{2}{(\cancel{1mg})}\ (1 tablet)}{(\cancel{0.5\ mg})}$$

$$(2)\ (1 tablet)$$

$$= 2\ tablets$$

So, the nurse will give 2 tablets of cogentin to the patient.

10) B

Doctor's Order: 2 Gm of Robaxin.

Label Relationship: 1 Gm per tablet or 1Gm/1 tablet or 1 tablet/1 Gm

Set Up: (To be Given Doctor's Order) (Right Relationship)

$$\frac{\overset{2}{(2\ \cancel{Gm})(1\ tablet)}}{(1\cancel{Gm})}$$

$$= (2)(1\ tablet)$$

$$= 2\ tablets$$

So, the nurse will give 2 tablets of Robaxin to the patient.

ADMINISTRATION OF LIQUID MEDICATIONS

Liquid medications are measured in volumes. The units for the volumes used in Nursing is cubic Centimeters or CC. This is the same as milliliters.

In Nursing, we deal with two forms of liquid medications. Liquid medications taken by mouth or liquid medications used as injectables.

LIQUID MEDICATIONS TAKEN BY MOUTH

We pour liquid medications into graduated cups.

We have to remember that the lower level of the liquid called the meniscus has to be at eye level for the accurately read volume.

When pouring liquid medications from bottles, we must put the hand around the label while we pour the medication. Make sure to immediately wipe any liquid drippings from the side of the bottle.

Table we must remember:

Milliliters (mls) = Cubic Centimeters (cc's) = (1/1,000) L=0.001L

1,000 cc (mls) = 1 Liter(L)

Now we are ready to administer medications in liquid form.

Example 1

The patient has a Gastrostomy tube (GT). The Doctor orders aceta-menophen (tylenol) 650 mg via the GT for a temperature greater than 101 degrees Fahrenheit every 6 hours Prn. Acetaminophen comes from the manufacturer as 325 mg in 5 cc. If the patient has a temperature of 101.6 degrees how many cc of medication will the nurse give the patient?

Answer

To be Given Doctor's order: 650 mg of Tylenol

Label Relationship: 325 mg in 5 cc or 5cc/325mg or 325 mg/5 cc

Set Up: (To be Given Doctor's order) (Right Relationship)

$$\frac{(\cancel{650}^{\,2} \text{ mg})(5\text{cc})}{(\cancel{325} \text{ mg})}$$
$$= (2 \times 5) \text{ cc}$$
$$= 10 \text{ cc}$$

So, the nurse will give 10 cc of Tylenol through the gastrostomy tube.

Example 2

The doctor wants you to give 200 mg. The label on the medication bottle reads 80 mg/2 ml. You would give-ml(s).

Answer

To be Given doctor's order: 200 mg

Label Relationship: 80 mg/2ml or 2ml/80 mg

Set up: (To be Given doctor's order) (Right Relationship)

$$\frac{(\cancel{200\ mg})^{5}(\cancel{2\ ml})^{1}}{(\cancel{80\ mg})}$$
$$(5)\,(1\ ml)$$
$$5\ ml$$

So. the nurse will give 5 mls of medication to the patient.

Example 3

The doctor wants you to give 600,000 units of heparin. The label reads 300,000 units/ml. You should give-ml(s).

Answer

To be Given doctor's order: 600,000 units of heparin.

Label Relationship: 300,000 units/1 ml or 1 ml/300,000 units

Ser up: (To be Given doctor's order) (Right Relationship)

$$\frac{(\overset{2}{\cancel{600,000 \text{ units}}}) (1 \text{ ml})}{(\underset{1}{\cancel{300,000 \text{ units}}})}$$

$$(2) (1 \text{ ml})$$
$$2 \text{ mls}$$

So, the nurse will give 2 cc or 2 mls of heparin to the patient.

Example 4

The doctor orders 4,000 units of heparin to be given to the patient. The label reads 10,000 units per ml. You should give-ml(s)

Answer

ANALYSIS

To be Given Doctor's order: 4,000units of heparin

Label Relation.:10,000units p per ml or 10,000units/1ml or 1ml/10,000units

Set Up: (To be Given Doctor's Order) (Label Relationship)

$$\frac{(4{,}000 \text{ units})(1 \text{ ml})}{(10{,}000 \text{ units})}$$

$$\frac{\overset{2}{(4{,}000 \text{ units})}(1 \text{ ml})}{\underset{5}{(10{,}000 \text{ units})}}$$

$$\frac{(2)(1 \text{ ml})}{5}$$

$$= 0.4 \text{ ml}$$

So, the nurse will give 0.4 ml of heparin to the patient.

NB/

Let us go through the strategy of algebra used here. This strategy is to change the fraction to a decimal. As we know in dividing with numbers that are factors of 10, we will just move the decimal point in the numerator.

For any fraction, the numerator is the top number and the denominator is the lower number.

For any fraction, when we multiply the denominator and the numerator with the same number, the value of the fraction remains the same.

The idea is to change the denominator to a factor of 10, i.e. 1,10,100,1,000

E.g. $\dfrac{(2)}{(5)}$

In the example here, we will multiply the denominator by 2. Here (5x2) = 10, which is a factor of 10.

The second step is to multiply the numerator with the same number. i.e.

(2x2) = 4

$\dfrac{(2x2)}{(5x2)}$

$\dfrac{(4)}{(10)}$

Since the denominator ends in only one zero, we move the decimal point which is after the 4 to the left only once, and we get, 0.4. This is because, the denominator which is 10, has only one zero.

So 4/5=0.4

Example 5

How many cc(ml) are in 2 L

Answer

ANALYSIS

To be Given: 2 L

Table Relationship: 1,000ml (cc)=1 Liter or 1L/1,000ml or 1,000ml/1L

Set up: (To be Given) (Table Relationship)

$$\frac{(2\cancel{L})\ (1,000ml)}{1\cancel{L}}$$
$$(2 \times 1,000)\ ml$$
$$2,000\ ml\ (cc)$$

So, there are 2,000 ce in 2 Liters

INJECTABLE LIQUID MEDICATIONS

Liquid medications can be given as injectables. Medications can be injected into the vein, into muscles, intradermal, or subcutaneous. The liquid medication is drawn into a syringe and the liquid injected in mls or cc's.

Example 1

The doctor orders Demerol (meperedine hydrochloride) for a patient in sickle cell anemia crisis. The doctor's order reads, Demerol 50 mg IMQ4H. The floor has Demerol labeled as 100 mg/ml. How many cc's of Demerol will the nurse give the patient when the patient complains of pain?

Answer

Doctor's order: 50 mg of Demerol

Label relationship: 100 mg/ml or 1ml/100 mg or 100mg per 1 ml

Ser up: (doctor's order) (label relationship)

$$\frac{(\overset{1}{\cancel{50mg}})(1ml)}{(\underset{2}{\cancel{100\ mg}})}$$

½ ml = 0.5 ml

OR

Multiplying numerator and denominator by 5,

we get,

$$\frac{(1 \times 5)}{(2 \times 5)} = \frac{5}{10}$$

$$= 0.5 \text{ ml}$$

= 5/10 = 0.5ml (moving the decimal point one step to the left, since the denominator 10 has only one zero).

So, the nurse will draw up 0.5 ml of Demerol into the syringe and give to the patient IM.

Example 2

For pain. the doctor orders dilaudid (hydromorphone hydrochloride). The doctor's order reads, give dilaudid 4 mg IM Q4H PRN for pain. Dilaudid comes from the manufacturer in tubex of 2 mg/ml. How many cc's of dilaudid will the nurse inject IM?

Answer

Doctor's order: 4 mg of dilaudid

Label Relationship: 2 mg/ml or 1 ml/2 mg or 1 mg per 2 ml

NB: Choose any label relationship that help you cancel the units you don't need. Here we will choose the relationship, 1 ml/2mg.

Ser up: (doctor's order) (Label Relationship)

$$\frac{(4 \, \cancel{mg})^{2} \, (1 \, ml)}{(2 \, \cancel{mg})_{1}}$$

$$\frac{(2)(1ml)}{2ml}$$

So, the nurse will give 2 cc or 2 ml of dilaudid injection to the patient when he complained of pain.

Example 3

Demerol has been ordered for a patient who is in severe pain. The doctor's order reads; Give demerol 50 mg IM every 4 hours for severe pain. Demerol is supplied as 50mg=1 cc. How many ml of demerol will the nurse give the patient when he complained of severe pain?

Answer:

Doctor's order: 50 mg

Label Relationship: 50mg=1cc or 50 mg/1cc or 1cc/50mg

Note: We can choose any of these relationships that help us do our calculations and cancellations effectively.

Set up: (To be Given doctor's order) (Right Relationship)

$$\frac{1}{\cancel{(50\ mg)}} \frac{(1\ cc)}{\cancel{(50\ mg)}}$$
$$\frac{1}{}$$
$$(1)\ (1cc)$$
$$1\ cc$$

So, the nurse will administer 1 cc of demerol to the patient 1M when he complained of severe pain.

Example 4

The doctor's order demerol reads; Give demerol 75 mg IM every 4 hours for pain PRN for pain. Demerol comes supplied as 50 mg per 1cc. When the patient complains of pain, how many cc of demerol will the doctor give to the patient when she complained of pain.

Answer:

Doctor's order: 75 mg of demerol

Supplier Relationship:50 mg=1cc or 50 mg/1cc or 1 cc/50mg

Ser Up: (doctor's order) (Right Relationship)

$$\frac{(\overset{3}{\cancel{75\ mg}})\ (1\ cc)}{(\underset{2}{\cancel{50\ mg}})}$$

$$= (\frac{3}{2}\ x1)\ cc$$

$$= \frac{3}{2}\ cc$$

or

$$\left(\frac{3}{2} \times \frac{5}{5}\right)\ cc = \frac{15}{10}\ cc$$

$$= 1.5\ cc$$

So the nurse will inject the patient with 1.5 cc of demerol when she complains of pain.

Example 5

The doctor's order reads Give demerol 25 mg IM for pain every 4 hours PRN. The demerol supplied at the unit is 100mg = 1 cc How many cc of demerol will the doctor give the patient when he complained of pain?

Answer:

Doctor's order: 25 mg

Label Relationship: 100 mg = 1cc

Set up: (Doctor's order) (Right Relationship)

$$\frac{\overset{1}{(\cancel{25\ mg})}\,(1cc)}{\underset{4}{(\cancel{100\ mg})}}$$

¼ cc = 0.25 cc

So the nurse will give 0.25 cc of demerol to the patient when she complained of pain.

QUESTIONS ON ADMINISTRATION OF LIQUID MEDICATION

Question 1

The doctor orders for the client to receive atropine sulfate 75 mg. The vial reads atropine sulfate 200mg=2cc. How much of this medication should the nurse administer to the client?

    a)   0.25 cc
    b)   0.50 cc
    c)   0.75 cc
    d)   1.25 cc

Question 2

The doctor ordered for the client to receive 250,000 units of penicillin. The available vial of the drug reads 2,000,000 units of penicillin diluted in 10 cc. How many cc will be administered to this client?

    a)   0.50 cc
    b)   0.75 cc
    c)   1.25 cc
    d)   2.50 cc

Question 3

The doctor orders 200 mg of docusate sodium (colace) to be given to a patient. The medication label reads: 100 mg in 5 cc. How many cc (mls) will the nurse give to the patient.

a) 5 cc
b) 10cc
c) 15 cc
d) 20 cc

Question 4

A six-year-old boy with a cardiac condition weighs forty-four pounds. He has been digitalized with 0.05 mg of digitoxin per kilogram of body weight. He is now receiving 1/4 of the dosage. How many milligrams of digitoxin will he be To be Given?

a) 0.25 mg
b) 1.4 mg
c) 1.0 mg
d) 0.75 mg

Question 5

The doctor has just started a patient on acyclovir. The patient is to receive 2 milliliters of acyclovir injection. Acyclovir is supplied 5 mg/ml. How many mg of acyclovir will the nurse give the patient?

a) 5 mg
b) 1 mg
c) 10 mg
d) 7.5 mg

Question 6

The doctor orders morphine sulfate for a patient post operatively. The order is Morphine sulfate 4 mg sq every 4hrs for pain. Morphine sulfate comes supplied as 5 mg/ml. When the patient complains of pain, how many milliliters of morphine sulfate will the nurse give to the patient?

a) 0.8 ml
b) 1.0 ml
c) 1.5 ml
d) 2.0 ml

Question 7

The doctor orders demerol be given to a patient in sickle cell crisis. The doctor's order is demerol 100 mg IM every 2 hours for severe pain. Demerol is supplied as 100 mg/ml. How many milliliters of demerol will the nurse give to this patient when he complains of pain?

a) 0.5 ml
b) 1.0 ml
c) 1.5 ml
d) 2.0 ml

Question 8

Oxymorphone Hydrochloride has been ordered for a patient in pain. The order reads, oxymorphone hydrochloride 3 mg every six hours. Oxymorphone hydrochloride is supplied as 1.5 mg/ml. How many milliliters will the nurse give the patient when she complains of pain?

a) 1.0 ml
b) 1.5 ml
c) 2.5 ml
d) 2.0 ml

Question 9

Papaverine has been ordered for a patient. The order is to give papaverine injection 60 mg every 12 hours. Papaverine is supplied as 30 mg/ml. How many milliliters of papaverine will the nurse give to the patient?

- a) 1 ml
- b) 2 ml
- c) 3 ml
- d) 4 ml

Question 10

The doctor orders Benadryl for a patient having insomnia. The order is for Benadryl 50 mg 1M. Benadryl comes supplied as 50 mg/ml. How many milliliters of Benadryl will the nurse give the patient when she complains of insomnia?

- a) 1 ml
- b) 2 ml
- c) 3 ml
- d) 4 ml

ADMINISTRATION OF INTRAVENOUS MEDICATIONS

This is a big part of medication administration.

Intravenous medications are infused directly into the veins. It can be either through a peripheral vein or through a central vein. In intravenous infusions we are concerned with the amount of fluid to be infused and the duration of time the fluid or the medication has to infuse.

We are also concerned about the drip chamber; Whether it is microdrip or a macrodrip. That will tell us the number of drops in a cc. Macrodrip chambers can release 12 or 15 drops in cc. Macrodrip chambers release 60 drops in a cc. Once we know the volume of fluid to be infused, time duration for infusion, and the drip factor, we are ready to set our drops per minute.

Noter We should also remember the following points:

1 hour - 60 minutes
60 seconds =1 minute
24 hours = 1 day
7 days =1 week
1 ml =1 cc = 15 or 16 minims = 15 or 16 drops
4 or 5 ml = 1 fluid dram = 1 tsp
60 or 65 mg - 1gr
30 or 32 ng = 1/2 gr
30 gm = 30 ml = 1 oz =2 tbsp

250 ml = 8 oz - 1 cup
454 gm = 1 lb
500 ml = 500 cc = 16 OZ = 1 pint
1 liter = 1000 ml = 32 OZ = 1 quart
1000g = 1 kg = 2.2 lb
0.6 g = 600 mg or 650 mg = 10 gr

We should be able to use any of these relationships and their combinations effectively.

Example 1

The rate of a certain IV solution is 100 ml/h. The drop factor of the IV tubing is 15 gtts/ml. What will be the gtts/min of this IV fluid?

Answer: Please note that our final answer will be in gtts/min.

With this in mind, and by using our general concept of solving medication calculations, our statement for the solution becomes:

$$\frac{\overset{25}{(\cancel{100\ ml})}\ \overset{1}{(15\ drops)}\ (1\ \cancel{hr})}{(1\ \cancel{hr})\ (\cancel{ml})\ (\cancel{60}\ mins)}$$

$$\frac{4}{25\ drops/min}$$

After cancellations, our final answer becomes, 25 drops/min.

Example 2

An order of 3,000 ml of IV fluid is to be infused over 24 hour period. The drop factor of the IV tubing is 10 gtts/ml. How many gtts/min will the IV fluid infuse?

Answer

To be Given: 3,000 ml to infuse over 24 hours.

Set up:

$$\frac{\overset{50}{(\cancel{3,000\ ml})}\ (10\ gtts)\ (1\ \cancel{hour})}{(24\ \cancel{h})\ (1\ \cancel{ml})\ (\cancel{60}\ mins)}$$
$$\underset{25\quad 5}{}$$

$$\frac{(\cancel{50})\ (\cancel{10})\ gtts}{(\cancel{24})\ min}$$
$$\underset{6}{}$$

$$\frac{(125\ gtts)}{6\ mins}$$
$$= 21\ gtts\ /min$$

38

Example 3

An IV solution of 500 mls is to be over 8 hours. The drop factor of the IV tubing is 60 gtts/ml. You should infuse the solution at---- gtts/min.

Answer:

To be Given: 500 mls over 8 hours

Set Up:
$$\frac{(500\ \text{ml})\ (60\ \text{gtts})\ (1\text{h})}{(8\text{h})\ (1\ \text{ml})\ (60\text{-mins})}$$

$$\frac{(500)\text{gtts}}{8\ \text{mins}}$$

$$=63\ \text{gtts/min}$$

or

63 gtts/min.

After cancellation, our answer becomes 62.5 gtts/min.

Since we don't have half of a drop, our final answer therefore becomes 63 gtts/min.

Note here carefully that: if the number after the decimal were to be 1, 2, 3, or 4, i.e., 1, .2, .3, or .4 our answer will be **62 gtts/min.**

Example 4

An IV fluid of 1,000 mls is to be infused at 150 ml/h. The fluid will be infused for how long?

To be Given 1,000 mls to be infused at 150 ml/h

Ser Up

$$\frac{(1,000 \text{ ml})(h)}{(150 \text{ ml})}$$
$$= 6.67 \text{ h}$$
$$= 7 \text{ hours}$$

So the fluid will be infused for 7 hours

Example 5

An IV fluid of 1,000 cc is to be infused at 125 cc/h. How many hours will you infuse this IV fluid?

Answer:

To be Given 1,000 cc to be infused at 125cc/h.

Ser Up

$$\frac{8}{(1,000 \text{ cc})(1 \text{ h})}{(125 \text{ cc})}$$
$$\frac{}{1}$$
$$(8)(1) \text{ h}$$
$$8 \text{ hours}$$

So the IV fluid will be infused for 4 hours.

QUESTIONS ON IV INFUSION

Question 1

A patient is to receive 3,000 ml (3 liters) of 5% Dextrose/Water within a 24-hour period. How many drops per minute should the nurse regulate the patient's intravenous fluid? (The dropper reads 10 gtts.= 1cc.)

a)   10 gtts/min
b)   21 gtts/min
c)   30 gtts/min
d)   40 cc/min

Question 2

The physician orders 1,500 cc of intravenous fluid to be given in 24 hours. The dropper reads 12 gtts= 1cc. The patient will receive how many drops per minute?

a)   8 gtts/minute
b)   13 gtts/minute
c)   20 gtts/minute
d)   32 gtts/minute

Question 3

The physician's order reads heparin sodium 25,000 units in 250 ml
5% dextrose in water to run continuously at a rate of 800 units per
hour by IV. The nurse sets the intravenous pump to how many ml
per hour?

a)   7 ml/h
b)   8 ml/h
c)   9 ml/h
d)   10 ml/h

Question 4

A physician's order reads 'haloperidol decanoate (Haldol) 175 mg
IM. The medication is available in 100 mg per ml. How many milliliters of the medication would a nurse draw into the syringe for
injection?

a)   1.5 ml
b)   1.8 ml
c)   1.9 ml
d)   1.25 ml

Question 5

A physician's order reads: tobramycin sulfate (nebcin), 75 mg IM
bid. The medication label reads: 10 mg/ml. A nurse prepares how
many millimeters to administer one dose?

a)   2.5 ml
b)   5.0 ml
c)   7.5 ml
d)   1.33 ml

Question 6

The physician's order reads: piperacillin sodium (pipracil), 650 mg IV every 6 hours. The medication label reads: 2 g and reconstitute with 5 ml of bacteriostatic water. The nurse prepares to draw up how many ml to administer one dose?

a)   0.62 ml
b)   1.0 ml
c)   1.63 ml
d)   5.0 ml

Question 7

The doctor's order reads: 'Give dobutamine chydrochloride(dobutrex) 5 mcg/kg/min.' Dobutamine comes reconstituted as 200 mg per 250ml solution of 5% dextrose in water. The patient weighs 110 pounds. At what rate (ml/hr) will the nurse set the infusion pump for the dobutamine drip?

a)   10 cc/h
b)   19 cc/h
c)   12 cc/h
d)   13 cc/h

Question 8

The physician's order for natrecor infusion is 0.01 Imcg/kg/min. The patient weighs 100 kg. Natrecor is reconstituted as 1.5 mg in 250 ml D5/0.9% Nacl. At what rate will the nurse set the infusion pump for the natrecor drip?

a)   10 cc/h
b)   11 cc/h
c)   2 cc/h
d)   13 cc/h

Question 9

The physicians order for the infusion of epinephrine drip is 0.0001 mg/kg/min. The patient weighs 100 kg. Epinephrine is reconstituted as 1mg in 100 cc of fluid. At what rate will the nurse set the infusion pump to deliver the correct amount of epinephrine?

a) 50 cc/h
b) 60 cc/h
c) 70 cc/h
d) 80 cc/h

Question 10

The doctor orders nitroglycerine drip for a patient as 5 mcg/min. Nitroglycerine is recostited as 10 mg in 100 cc of 5% dextrose in water. At what rate will the nurse set the IV pump at to deliver the correct amount of nitroglycerine?

a) 2 cc/h
b) 3 cc/h
c) 4 cc/h
d) 5 cc/h

ANSWERS TO LIQUID
MEDICATION QUESTIONS

1/ C

ILLUSTRATION

Doctor's order: 75 mg
Label Relationship: 200 mg = 2 cc

Set up: (doctor's order) (Label Relationship)

$$\frac{\overset{3}{\cancel{(75\ mg)}}\ \overset{1}{(2\ cc)}}{\underset{\underset{4}{8}}{\cancel{(200\ mg)}}}$$

¾ cc = 0.75 cc

So, the nurse will administer 0.75 CC of atropine sulfate to the patient.

2/C

Doctor's order: 250,000 units of penicillin.
Label relationship: 2,000,000 units of penicillin in 10 cc

Set up: (doctor's order) (Label Relationship)

$$\frac{\cancel{25}\,5}{\cancel{(250,000}\,\text{units})(\cancel{10}\,\text{cc})}{(\cancel{2,000,0000}\,\text{units})}$$

$$\frac{\cancel{20}}{4}$$

$$5/4 \text{ cc} = 1.25 \text{ cc}$$

Or

$$\frac{5 \times 25}{4 \times 25}$$

$$\frac{125}{100}$$

$$= 1.25 \text{ cc}$$

No the nurse will administer 1.25 cc of penicillin to the patient.

3/ B

Doctor's order: 200 mg of colace
Label Relationship: 100 mg in 5 cc.

Set up:(doctor's order) (Label Relationship)

$$\frac{(\overset{2}{\cancel{200\ mg}})\ (5\ cc)}{\underset{1}{(\cancel{100\ mg})}}$$

$$(2)\ (5)cc$$
$$= 10\ cc$$

So the nurse will administer 10 cc of colace to the patient.

4/ A

Doctor's order: 0.05 mg per kg of body weight
Patient's weight: 44 pounds
Note: 2.2 pounds (2.2 lbs) = 1 kg

Since we want the answer in kg, we have to change our weight in lbs to kg. So that adds one more step to our set up.
(Doctor's order) (Label Relationship) (Others)

$$\frac{(0.05\ mg)\ (44\ \cancel{lbs})\ (1\ \cancel{kg})}{(1\ \cancel{kg})\ (2.2\ \cancel{lbs})}$$

$$\frac{(0.05\ mg)\ (44x10)}{(2.2x10)}$$

$$\frac{(0.05\ mg)\ (\overset{20}{\cancel{440}})}{\underset{1}{\cancel{22}}}$$

$$(0.05\ mg)\ (20)$$

$$= 1.0\ mg$$

If now the patient receives 1/4 the dosage, The nurse will administer
¼ x 1 mg = 0.25 mg of digitoxin.

5/ C

Doctor's order: 2 ml
Label Relationship: 5 mg/ml
Set up:(doctor's order) (Label Relationship)

$$\frac{(2 \text{ ml}) \ (5 \text{ mg})}{(\text{ml})}$$

$$(2) \ (5 \text{ mg})$$
$$= 10 \text{ mg}$$

So the nurse will administer 10 mg of acyclovir to the patient.

6/ A

Doctor's order: 4 mg
Label Relationship: 5 mg/ml
set up (doctor's order) (Label Relationship)

$$\frac{(4 \text{ mg}) \ (\text{ml})}{(5 \text{ mg})}$$

$$= 4/5 \text{ ml} = 0.8 \text{ ml}$$

So the nurse will administer 0.8 ml of medication to the patient.

7/ B

Doctor's order: 100 mg
Label Relationship: 100 mg/ml
Set Up: (Doctor's order) (Label Relationship)

$$\frac{(\cancel{100}\ \cancel{mg})(1\ ml)}{(\cancel{100}\ \cancel{mg})}$$

$$= 1\ ml$$

So the nurse will give 1 ml of demerol injection to the patient in sickle cell crisis

8/ D

Doctor's order: 3 mg
Label Relationship: 1.5 mg/ml
Set Up: (doctor's order) (Label Relationship)

$$\frac{\overset{2}{\cancel{(3\ mg)}}\ (1\ ml)}{(\cancel{1.5\ mg})}$$

$$= 2.0\ ml$$

So nurse will give 2 ml of medication to the patient

9/ B

Doctor's order: 60 mg
Label Relationship: 30 mg/ml
Set Up (doctor's order) (Label Relationship)

$$\frac{(\overset{2}{\cancel{60\ mg}})(1\ ml)}{(\underset{1}{\cancel{30\ mg}})}$$

$$(2)ml = 2\ ml$$

So the nurse will give 2 ml of medication to the patient

10/ C

Doctor's order: 150 mg
Label Relationship: 50 mg/ml
Set Up (doctor's order) (Label Relationship)

$$\frac{(\overset{3}{\cancel{150\ mg}})(1\ ml)}{(\underset{1}{\cancel{50\ mg}})}$$

$$= 3ml$$

So the nurse will give 3 ml of medication to the patient.

ANSWERS TO INTRAVENOUS INFUSION MEDICATIONS AND DRIPS

1/ B

Doctor's order: 3,000 ml in 24 hours
Dropper Relationship: 10 gtts = 1 cc

Set up: (Doctor's order) (Dropper Relationship) (Others)

It should be noted here that the others will be relationships we can get from tables. Our answer must be in gtts/min. So we have to use any right relationship we know of to help us arrive at this answer. This is what we represent in the set up as "others".

Here our others will be: 1 hour (1h) - 60 minutes (mins)

Our Set up then becomes:

$$\frac{\overset{50}{\cancel{(3,000\ ml)}}\ (10\ gtts)\ \cancel{(1\ h)}}{\underset{1}{(24\ \cancel{h})\ (1\ ml)\ \cancel{60\ min})}}$$

20.83333gtts/min = 21 gtts/min

Since in reality, there is nothing like a fraction of a drop, and 0.8 is greater than 0.5, Our answer becomes 21 gtts/min

2/ B

Physician's order: 1,500 cc to be given in 24 hours
Drop Relationship: 12 gtts = 1cc
Set Up: (Physician's order) (drop relationship) (others)

$$\frac{\overset{25}{(\cancel{1,500cc})} \overset{1}{(\cancel{12}\text{ gtts})} (1h)}{\underset{2}{(\cancel{24\,h})} (\cancel{cc}) \underset{1}{(\cancel{60}\text{ min})}}$$

25/2 gtts/min = 12.5gtts/min
= 13 gtts/min

be the patient will receive a fluid of 13 drops per minute

3/ B

Physician's order: 800 units per hour
Label Relationship: 25,000 units in 250 ml 5% dextrose
Set up: (Physician's order) (Label Relationship) (others)

$$\frac{\overset{8}{(\cancel{800\text{ units}})} \overset{1}{(\cancel{250}\text{ ml})}}{(1h) (\cancel{25,000\text{ units}})}$$
$$\frac{\cancel{100}}{\cancel{8}\text{-ml/h}}$$

= 8 ml/h

So the nurse will set the infusion pump at a rate of 8ml/h

4/ B

Physician's order: 175 mg
Label Relationship: 100 mg/ml
Set up:(Physician's order) (Label Relationship)

$$\frac{(\overset{7}{\cancel{175\ mg}})\ (1\ ml)}{(\underset{4}{\cancel{100\ mg}})}$$

7/4 ml=1.75 or 1.80 ml

So the nurse will give 1.80 ml of haldol to the patient

5/ C

Physician's order: 75 mg
Label Relationship: 10 mg/ml
Set up: (Physician's order) (Label Relationship)

$$\frac{(75\ \cancel{mg})\ (1\ ml)}{(10\ \cancel{mg})}$$

$$\frac{75\ ml}{10}$$

7.5 ml

So the nurse will administer 7.5 ml of tobramycin to the patient.

6/ C

Physician's order: 650 mg IV in 6 hours
Label Relationship: 2 g with 5 ml
Set up (Physician's order) (Label Relationship) (other

$$\frac{\overset{325}{\cancel{(650\ mg)}}\ (5\ ml)\ \cancel{(1\ gm)}}{\underset{1}{\cancel{(2\ gm)}\ (1,000\ \cancel{mg})}}$$

$$=\frac{1,625\ ml}{1,000} = 1,625/1000ml$$

$$= 1.63\ ml$$

So the nurse will draw up 1.63 ml of the medication.

7/ B

Doctor's order: 5 mcg/kg/min
Label Relationship: 200 mg per 250 ml
Weight of patient: 110 pounds (110 lbs)
Set up: (Doctor's order) (Label Relationship) (others)

$$\frac{(1\ \cancel{kg})\cancel{(110\ lbs)}(1)(5\ \cancel{mg})(250\ ml)\cancel{(60\ mins)}\cancel{(1mg)}}{\cancel{(2.2\ lbs)}\cancel{(kg(min)}(200mg)(1h)\cancel{(1,000mg)}}$$

$$\frac{1875\ ml}{100h} = 18.75ml/h$$

$$= 19\ ml\ /\ h$$

So the infusion pump will be set at 19 ml/h

8/ A

Doctor's order 0.01 mcg/kg/min
Reconstitution relationship: 1.5 mg in 250 ml D5/0.9% NaCl
Wight of patient 100 kg
Set Up: (Doctor's order) (Reconstitution Relation) (others)

$$\frac{(0.01\text{mg}) \overset{1}{(100\text{Kg})} \overset{1}{(250\text{ cc})} (60\text{ mins}) (1\text{mg})}{(\text{kg})(\text{min})(1.5\text{ mg})(1{,}000\text{ mcg})(1\text{h})}$$

$$\frac{\overset{4}{60\text{cc}}}{6} = 10\text{cc/h}$$

So the nurse will set the infusion pump at 10cc/h

9/ B

Physician's order: 0.0001 mg/kg/min
Label order; 1 mg in 100 cc
Weight of patient: 100 kg

Set up: (Physician's order) (Label Relationship) (others)

$$\frac{(100\text{ kg}) \overset{1}{(0.0001\text{mg})} (100\text{cc}) (60\text{ min})}{(1\text{ mg}) (\text{kg}) (\text{min}) (1\text{h})}$$

60cc/h

So the nurse will set the pump at 60 cc/h

10/ B

Doctor's order: 5mcg/min
Reconstituted Relationship: 10 mg in 100 cc of 5%
Dextrose in water.
Set up:

$$\left(\frac{(Doctor's\ order)}{(Reconstituted\ Relationship)} \right)$$

$$\frac{(5\ \text{mcg})\ (100\ cc)\ (60\ \text{min})\ (1\ \text{mg})}{(\text{min})\ (10\ \text{mg})\ (1h)\ (1,000\ \text{mcg})}$$

$$\frac{30cc}{10h}$$

$$=3\ cc/h$$

So the nurse will set the infusion pump to deliver 3 cc/h

GENERAL QUESTIONS ON MEDICATION ADMINISTRATION

Answers starts on page 76

SET 1

1. Which of these abbreviations indicates that a drug is to be administered a regularly spaced intervals during each 24-hour period?

   A. q8h
   B. qid
   C. q6h, prn

2. How many milligrams are equivalent to 0.055 grams?

   A. 5.5
   B. 55
   C. 550

3. Which of these doses is the smallest?

   A. 0.2 gm
   B. 0.02 mg
   C. 20 mg

4. A 2 ml syringe illustrated below contains the amount of solution indicated by the arrows. How many milliliters of solution does the syringe contain?

A. 1.2
B. 1.4
C. 1.6

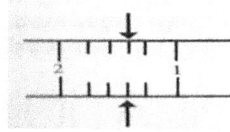

5. A child is to receive amoxicillin(amoxil) 60 mg PO. The medication is supplied as an oral suspension containing 125 mg per ml. How many milliliters should the child receive?

A. 1.2
B. .48
C. 25

6. A patient is to receive cephalexin(keflex) 1 gm po. Keflex is available as 500 mg tablets. How many tablets should be administered?

A. 2
B. 3
C. 4

7. A patient is to receive cyanocobalamin (vitamin B12) 40 mcg IM. Vitamin B12 is available in 100 mcg per ml. How many milliliters should be administered?

A. 0.5
B. 0.4
C. 3.0

8. Penicillin G sodium for injection contains 500,000 units per milliliter. How many units would there be in 5.0 ml?

   A. 2.5 million
   B. 100,000
   C. million

9. A patient is to receive meperidine (demerol) hydrochloride 100 mg and atropine sulfate 0.4 mg IM preoperatively. Demerol is available in a prepackaged syringe containing 100 mg per ml. Atropine is available in a vial containing 0.4 mg per ml. If the two drugs were combined in the same syringe for administration, how many milliliters would be given?

   A. 1.5
   B. 2.0
   C. 2.5

10. A patient is to receive 1000 ml of IV fluid in 8 hours. The infusion pump should be set to deliver how many milliliters per hour?

   A. 100
   B. 120
   C. 125

11. A patient is to receive 500 ml of IV fluid during a 21/2 hour period. The intravenous setup delivers 15 drops per milliliter. The drip mechanism should be regulated to deliver approximately how many drops per minute?

   A. 40
   B. 50
   C. 60

12. A patient is to receive 1,000 ml of IV solution over 8 hours. Four later. 600 ml remain. The infusion set delivers 12 drops per milliliter To receive the remaining fluid within the prescribed time period. the ser should deliver how many drops per minute?

    A. 10
    B. 20
    C. 30

13. A patient is to receive gentamicin sulfate (Garamycin) 100 mg IV in 100 ml diluent over one hour. The intravenous setup delivers 15 drops per milliliter. How many drops per minute should the patient receive?

    A. 35
    B. 65
    C. 25

14. A patient is to receive digoxin (Lanoxin) 0.5 mg IV. Lanoxin is available in il prepackaged syringe containing 0.5 mg per 2 ml. How many milliliters should be administered?

    A. 1.0 ml
    B. 2.0 ml
    C. 3.0 ml

15. A U-100 syringe is illustrated below. The arrow indicates the level to which the syringe has been filled with insulin injection (Regular Insulin) labeled 100U per ml. How many units of insulin are in the syringe?

    A. 2.3
    B. 33
    C. 2.6

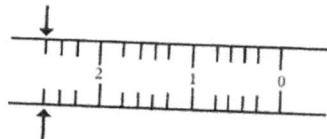

SET 2

1. Which of these abbreviations indicates that a drug is to be administered at regularly spaced intervals during each 24-hour period?

   A. q8h, prn
   B. q6h
   C. tid, pc

2. How many grams are equivalent to 3 milligrams?

   A. 0.003
   B. 0.03
   C. 0.3

3. Which of the following doses is the largest?

   A. 0.4 gm
   B. 4 mg
   C. .04 mg

4. Forty milliliters are equivalent to how many liters?

   A. 0.004
   B. 0.04
   C. 0.444

5. A child is to receive 400 mg of erythromycin(erythrocin). The medication is supplied as an oral suspension containing 200 mg per 5 ml. How many milliliters should the child receive?

   A. 2.0
   B. 5.0
   C. 10.0

6. Sulfisoxazole (Gantrisin) 3 gm is ordered for a patient. Gantrisin is available in 600 mg tablets. How many tablets should be administered to the patient?

   A. 3
   B. 4
   C. 5

7. Betamethasone sodium phosphate 6 mg is prescribed for a patient. The medication is supplied as a solution for injection containing 3 mg per milliliter. Approximately how many milliliters should the patient receive?

   A. 1
   B. 2
   C. 3

8. A patient is to receive 400,000 units of penicillin G potassium intramuscularly. The penicillin G potassium suspension contains 1 million units per milliliter. How many milliliters should the patient receive?

   A. 0.4
   B. 0.5
   C. 0.75

9. A patient is to receive 0.6 mg of digoxin (lanoxin) intravenously. Lanoxin is available in ampules containing 0.3 mg per milliliter. How many milliliters should be administered?

   A. 0.5
   B. 1.0
   C. 2.0

10. A patient is to receive 500,000 units of penicillin G procaine suspension (Wycillin). Wycillin is supplied 600,000 units per 1.2 milliliters. How many milliliters should the patient receive?

    A. 1.0
    B. 0.4
    C. 1.6

11. A patient weighs 132 lb (60 kg). The patient is to receive vin-blastine sulfate (velban) 0.15 mg per kg intravenously. How much Velban should be given?

    A. 4 mg
    B. 9 mg
    C. 18.9 mg

12. AU-100 insulin syringe is illustrated below. The arrow indicates the level to which the syringe has been filled with regular insulin labeled "100 U per ml". How many units of insulin are in the syringe?

    A. A/ 1.4
    B. B/ 14
    C. C/ 24

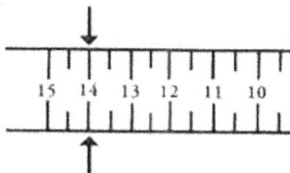

13. A patient is to receive 1,000 ml of fluids intravenously during a 24- hour period. The intravenous setup delivers 60 drops per milliliter. Approximately how many drops per minute should the drip mechanism be regulated to deliver.

    A. 40
    B. 41
    C. 42

14. A patient is to receive 480 ml intravenous fluids during a three-hour period. The intravenous setup delivers 15 drops per milliliter. The drip mechanism should be regulated to deliver how many drops per minute?

    A. 40
    B. 4.5
    C. 5

15. A patient is to receive 500 mg of cefazolin sodium (Kefzol) intravenously in 100 ml of 5% dextrose solution in two hours. The intravenous ser delivers 60 microdrops per milliliter. How many microdrops of the medication should be administered each minute?

    A. 40
    B. 50
    C. 60

SET 3

1. Which of these abbreviations indicate that a drug is to be administered twice a day during waking hours?

   A. q12h
   B. b.i.d.
   C. q.i.d.

2. How many milligrams are equivalent to 0.055 grams?

   A. 5.5
   B. 55
   C. 550

3. Which of these doses is the smallest?

   A. 0.4 Gm
   B. 0.04 mg
   C. 40 mg

4. A patient is to receive 500 mg of Penicillin G. PO. The medication is supplied as an oral suspension containing 250 mg per 10 ml. How many milliliters should the patient receive?

   A. 20
   B. 4.8
   C. 30

5. A patient is to receive 600 mg of a medication in a 24-hour period. The drug is to be given q6hrs. How many milligrams will be given for each dose?

   A. 160
   B. 150
   C. 260

6. A patient is to receive 30,000 units of heparin sodium IV push. The heparin is supplied in 10,000 u/ml. How many milliliters should a nurse administer?

    A. 0.5
    B. 2.5
    C. 3.0

7. A patient is to receive 1,200 ml of IV fluid in 3 hours. The infusion should be set for how many ml/hr?

    A. 400
    B. 300
    C. 350

8. A patient is to receive dopamine 100mg/200 ml D5W at the intravenous infusion rate of 1 mcg/Kg/min. The patient weighs 80 Kg. How many cc/hr should the patient receive?

    A. 11
    B. 12
    C. 9.6

9. A patient who weighs 20 Kg is to receive 5 mg/Kg/day of gentamycin sulfate(Garamycin) intravenously in divided doses q8hrs. The patient should receive how many milligrams of Garamycin with each dose?

    A. 30
    B. 33.3
    C. 3.33

10. A patient is to receive 1000 cc of IV fluid during a 5-hour period. the intravenous setup delivers 60 micro drops per milliliter. The drip mechanism should be regulated to deliver approximately how many microdrops per minute?

    A. 100
    B. 200
    C. 300

11. A patient is to receive 500 cc of IV solution over 5 hours. Three hours later, 300 cc remain. The infusion set delivers 12 drops per milliliter To receive the remaining fluid within the prescribed time period, the set should deliver how many drops per minute?

    A. 20
    B. 30
    C. 40

12. A patient is to receive 250 mg of Solu-Medrol IV push. Solu-Medrol is available in 125 mg/2cc vials. How many milliliters should be administered?

    A. 4.0
    B. 4.5
    C. 5.0

SET 4

1. Penicillin G benzathene (Bacillin) is available in prefilled syringes containing 1 million u/ml. If 250,000u of Bacillin is ordered for a client, how many milliliters should a nurse administer.

    A.   1
    B.   2
    C.   3
    D.   0.25

2. A nurse should recognize that a microdrip intravenous administration set is designed to administer how many drops of solution per milliliter.

    A.   12
    B.   15
    C.   60
    D.   10

3. A client who weighs 88 lbs (40 kg) is to receive dopamine hydrochloride (Intropin) at the rate of 2 mcg/kg/min. A nurse mixes 400 mg of Intropin in 250 ml of intravenous solution. The nurse should set the infusion pump to deliver how many milliliters per hour?

    A.   1
    B.   2
    C.   3
    D.   4

4. A client is to receive intravenous fluids at 100 ml/h. The infusion has been running for 3 hours and the client has received 400 ml of fluid. The infusion is running

   A. 1 hour behind schedule
   B. 30 minutes behind schedule
   C. 2 hours ahead of schedule
   D. 1 hour ahead of schedule

5. A client is to receive 10,000 units of heparin sodium. The heparin is supplied in 10,000 u/ml. How many milliliters should a nurse administer?

   A. 1
   B. 2
   C. 3
   D. 4

6. A client who weighs 60 kg is to receive 30 units/kg/hr of a medication as a continuous infusion. The intravenous solution contains 30,000 unite of the drug per 250 ml. The infusion pump should be set to deliver approximately how many milliliters per hour?

   A. 14
   B. 15
   C. 16
   D. 17

7. A client who weighs 20 kg is to receive 12 mg/kg/day of genta-
    micin sulfate (Garamycin) intravenously in divided doses q6h.
    The client should receive how many milligrams of Garamycin
    with each dose.

    A. 40
    B. 50
    C. 60
    D. 70

8. A client is to receive dobutamine hydrochloride (dobutrex) at
    the intravenous infusion rate of 2 mcg/kg/min. The patient
    weighs 80 he How many micrograms should the client receive
    in 5 minutes?

    A. 800
    B. 200
    C. 250
    D. 300

9. A client is to receive magnesium sulfate at the rate of 1 gm/hr. If
    10 gm of magnesium sulfate is placed in 100 ml of D5W, how
    many milliliters per hour will the client receive?

    A. 7
    B. 8
    C. 9
    D. 10

10. A patient is to receive 500 mg of a medication in a 12-hour period. The medication is to be given q6h. How many milligrams will be given for each dose?

   A. 150
   B. 200
   C. 250
   D. 300

11. Codeine liquid 15 mg is prescribed for a client. Codeine liquid is available as 15 mg/4 ml. How many milliliters should a nurse give?

   A. 1
   B. 2
   C. 3
   D. 4

12. A patient is to receive 500 mg of cephalexin (keflex) IV. The drug is diluted in 50 cc of D5W and is run over 30 minutes. Microdrip tubing (60 Microdrops/ml) is used. How many microdrops per minute should the nurse regulate the infusion set to deliver?

   A. 100
   B. 150
   C. 200
   D. 250

ANSWERS TO GENERAL QUESTIONS

SET 1
1) A
2) B
3) B
4) B
5) B
6) A
7) B
8) A
9) B
10) 1C
11) 1B
12) 1C
13) 1C
14) 1B
15) 1C

SET 2
1) B
2) A
3) A
4) B
5) C
6) C
7) B
8) A

9) C
10) 1A
11) 1B
12) 1B
13) 1C
14) 1A
15) 1B

SET 3

1) B
2) B
3) B
4) A
5) B
6) C
7) A
8) C
9) B
10) 1B
11) 1B
12) 1A

SET 4

1) D
2) C
3) C
4) D
5) A
6) B
7) C
8) A
9) D
10) 1C
11) 1D
12) 1A

ABOUT NURSING CALCULATIONS

I stumbled upon this method of medication calculation during an exam I took at Columbia Presbyterian Hospital in Manhattan, New York City. I did not know I was going to take an exam, so I did not revise the many numerous formulae of nursing calculations. At that moment my back was against the wall.

That would mean total failure for me. So, I looked in the air, put my head down and came up with this method. I tried it and it worked. Since then, I have tried it in all the exams I took in nursing and it worked wonders for every single problem. I decided to share this method which I hope will simplify medication calculations for all nurses and give them the peace of mind to care and free them of the precious time they need to take care of their patients.

My dream is that this method of nursing calculations in addition with the digital age will make nursing calculations for all nurses more fun and easier.